Australian Shepherd Training Book for First Time Owners

TATE SKINNER

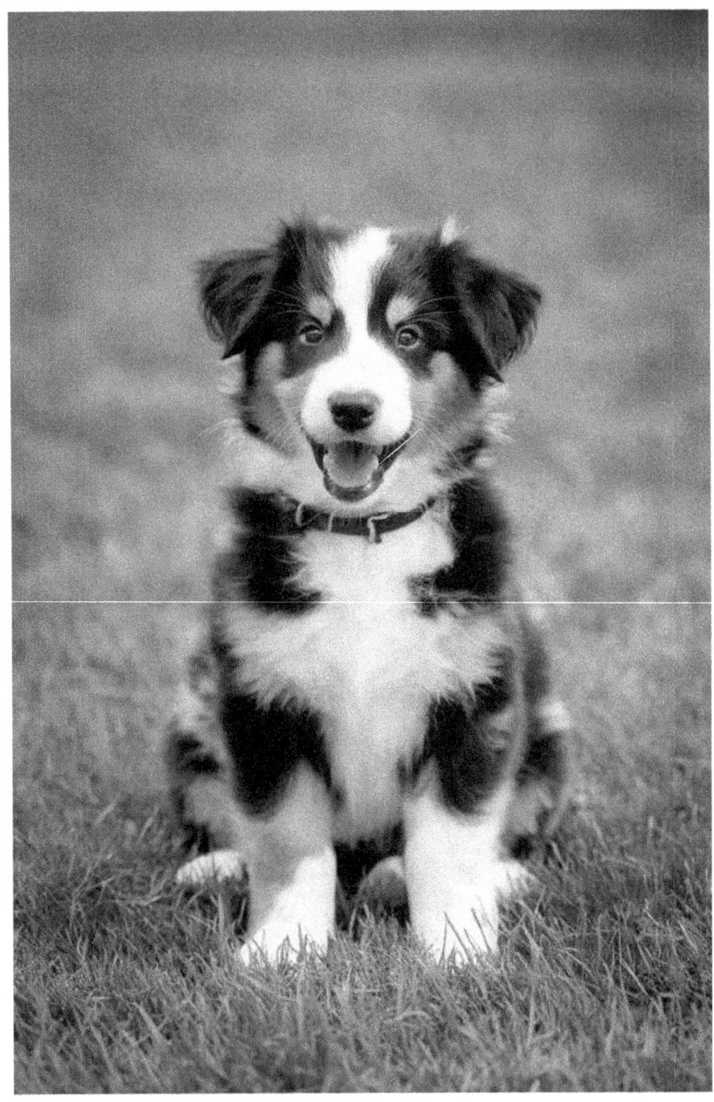

Copyright © 2024

by TATE SKINNER

Table of Contents

Introduction

Welcome to the World of Australian Shepherds

The Appeal of Australian Shepherds

History and Origin

The Australian Shepherd, affectionately known as the "Aussie," is a breed with a rich history and intriguing origins that contribute to its widespread appeal.

> **Misleading Name**: Despite its name, the Australian Shepherd was actually developed in the United States. The breed's ancestors, including various types of working collies, arrived in America via Australia, leading to the name "Australian Shepherd."

Development in the United States: In the late 19th and early 20th centuries, ranchers in the western United States sought a versatile herding dog. They selectively bred dogs for intelligence, work ethic, and agility. This resulted in the Australian Shepherd we know today.

Role on Ranches: Aussies quickly became indispensable on ranches, herding livestock and assisting with various tasks. Their ability to work long hours in challenging conditions earned them a reputation as one of the best working breeds.

Recognition: The Australian Shepherd was officially recognized by the American Kennel Club (AKC) in 1993. Its popularity has grown steadily, thanks to its exceptional skills and charming personality.

Unique Traits and Characteristics

Australian Shepherds possess several unique traits and characteristics that make them stand out among dog breeds:

Intelligence: Aussies are renowned for their high intelligence. They excel in obedience training, agility, and problem-solving tasks. This intelligence requires regular mental stimulation to prevent boredom.

Energy and Stamina: Bred for herding, Australian Shepherds have boundless energy and stamina. They thrive in active households where they can participate in regular physical activities such as hiking, running, and playing fetch.

Work Ethic: Their strong work ethic makes Aussies highly trainable and eager to please. They are often used in various roles, including search and rescue, therapy, and as service dogs.

Loyalty and Affection: Australian Shepherds form strong bonds with their families. They are known for their loyalty and affectionate nature, often seeking to be close to their owners and participating in family activities.

Protective Instincts: While generally friendly, Aussies can be protective of their families and territory. Early socialization is crucial to ensure they are well-mannered and confident around strangers.

Herding Instincts: Even if not used for herding, many Australian Shepherds display herding behaviors such as nipping at heels and circling. Channeling this instinct through appropriate training and activities is essential.

Preparing for Your Australian Shepherd

Understanding the Breed

Before bringing an Australian Shepherd into your home, it's important to understand the breed's specific needs and characteristics:

Exercise Requirements: Australian Shepherds need significant physical activity to stay happy and healthy. Aim for at least one to two hours of vigorous exercise daily, including walks, playtime, and mentally stimulating games.

Mental Stimulation: Their intelligence demands regular mental stimulation. Puzzle toys, training sessions, and interactive games are great ways to keep their minds engaged.

Socialization: Early and continuous socialization is vital. Expose your Aussie to various environments, people, and other animals to ensure they develop into well-rounded, confident adults.

Training: Consistent, positive reinforcement training is essential. Start with basic obedience commands and gradually introduce more advanced training to challenge their intellect.

Health Considerations: Australian Shepherds are generally healthy, but they can be prone to specific genetic conditions such as hip dysplasia, eye disorders, and epilepsy. Regular veterinary check-ups and a healthy diet are crucial for their well-being.

Essential Supplies and Equipment

Preparing your home for an Australian Shepherd involves gathering the necessary supplies and equipment to ensure their comfort and safety:

- **Crate**: A sturdy, appropriately sized crate provides a safe space for your puppy and aids in house training.
- **Bedding**: Comfortable bedding is essential for your Aussie's rest. Choose durable, washable materials.
- **Food and Water Bowls**: Stainless steel or ceramic bowls are ideal, as they are easy to clean and do not harbor bacteria.
- **High-Quality Dog Food**: Consult your veterinarian for recommendations on a balanced diet suitable for Australian Shepherds. Quality dog food supports their high energy levels and overall health.
- **Collar and Leash**: A durable collar and leash are essential for walks and training sessions. Consider a harness for added control during walks.
- **Identification Tags**: Ensure your Aussie has ID tags with your contact information in case they get lost.
- **Grooming Supplies**: Regular grooming helps maintain your Aussie's coat and overall

health. Essential supplies include a brush, comb, nail clippers, and ear cleaning solution.

- **Toys**: Provide a variety of toys to keep your Australian Shepherd mentally stimulated and entertained. Chew toys, puzzle toys, and fetch toys are excellent choices.
- **Training Tools**: Invest in basic training tools such as treats, a clicker, and training guides to support your training efforts.
- **First Aid Kit**: A pet-specific first aid kit is useful for addressing minor injuries and emergencies.

By understanding the breed's characteristics and preparing adequately, you'll be ready to welcome an Australian Shepherd into your home, setting the stage for a fulfilling and rewarding relationship with your new furry friend.

Chapter 1

Getting Started with Your Australian Shepherd

Choosing the Right Puppy

Breeders vs. Adoption

Breeders:

When deciding to purchase an Australian Shepherd puppy from a breeder, it is essential to ensure the breeder adheres to high ethical standards. Here's how to navigate this process effectively:

- **Research and Recommendations:** Utilize breed club directories and seek referrals from veterinarians and other dog owners. The ASCA and AKC are reputable sources.

- **Visit the Breeder:** Arrange a visit to inspect the breeding environment. Clean, spacious, and hygienic living conditions are indicators of a responsible breeder.
- **Ask Questions:** Inquire about the health history of the breeding pair, including genetic tests for common Australian Shepherd health issues such as hip dysplasia, eye conditions, and epilepsy. Documentation should be readily available.
- **Meet the Parents:** Observing the puppy's parents can provide insights into your future dog's temperament and size.
- **Health Guarantees:** Ensure the breeder offers health guarantees, typically covering genetic disorders, and be clear on the terms of any return policy.

Adoption:

Adopting an Australian Shepherd can be an immensely rewarding experience. Here's a guide to adopting successfully:

- **Rescue Organizations**: Many organizations focus on rehoming Australian Shepherds. Websites like Petfinder or specific breed rescues are excellent starting points.
- **Shelters**: Local shelters often have a variety of dogs, including Australian Shepherds or mixes. Visit multiple times to find a dog that fits your lifestyle.
- **Behavioral Assessments:** Most rescues perform behavioral evaluations. Discuss any concerns with the staff to understand the dog's temperament and any special needs.
- **Health Check:** Ensure the dog has been vet-checked, vaccinated, and neutered/spayed. Ask for medical records and any known history.

What to Look for in a Healthy Puppy

Selecting a healthy Australian Shepherd puppy involves careful observation and interaction. Here are some specific aspects to focus on:

- **Bright Eyes and Clean Ears**: Look for clear, bright eyes free from discharge, and clean ears without odor or redness, which could indicate infections.
- **Shiny Coat**: The coat should be soft, shiny, and free of parasites. Check for skin issues, bald patches, or signs of excessive scratching.
- **Active and Alert**: Healthy puppies are curious and playful. They should respond to stimuli, such as noises or movement, and engage in play with littermates.
- **Solid Build**: The puppy should have a sturdy build, moving freely without signs of limping or pain.
- **Breathing**: Check for steady, quiet breathing without coughing, wheezing, or nasal discharge.
- **Stool Check**: Observing the puppy's stool can provide insights into their digestive health. It should be firm and well-formed.

Bringing Your Puppy Home

Puppy-Proofing Your Home

Creating a safe environment for your Australian Shepherd puppy is crucial. Here are detailed steps to puppy-proof your home:

- **Secure Hazards**: Remove or secure potential hazards such as electrical cords, household chemicals, and small objects that could be swallowed. Use baby gates to block off areas that are not puppy-safe.
- **Safe Space**: Designate a specific area for your puppy, such as a crate or a puppy-proofed room. This space should include a comfortable bed, water, and toys. It will serve as a secure retreat and aid in house training.
- **Outdoor Safety**: Ensure your yard is secure with a fence high enough to prevent escapes. Remove toxic plants and

check for any sharp objects or gaps in the fence.

- **Chew Toys:** Provide a variety of chew toys to satisfy your puppy's teething needs and to prevent them from chewing on furniture or other household items.

First Days and Nights: Setting Expectations

The initial days with your new puppy are foundational for establishing routines and building trust. Here's how to manage this transition effectively:

- **Introducing the Crate**: Start crate training immediately. Place the crate in a quiet, familiar area. Make it inviting with comfortable bedding and a favorite toy. Use treats and positive reinforcement to encourage your puppy to see the crate as a safe space.
- **Establish a Routine**: Consistency is key. Establish regular times for feeding, potty

breaks, play, and sleep. This helps your puppy understand what to expect and reduces anxiety.

- **Feeding Schedule**: Feed your puppy at consistent times each day to regulate their digestion and facilitate house training. Consult your vet for a diet plan appropriate for your puppy's age and breed-specific needs.
- **Potty Training**: Take your puppy outside frequently, especially after meals, playtime, and naps. Praise and reward your puppy for successful potty breaks outside. Consistency and positive reinforcement are crucial. Use a specific spot in the yard to help your puppy associate the area with potty time.
- **Nighttime Adjustments**: Your puppy may feel anxious during the first few nights. Place the crate near your bed to provide comfort and reassurance. Expect some whining or crying, but avoid taking the puppy out unless it's for a scheduled potty

break. Gradually, your puppy will adjust to the new routine.

Establishing Basic Training Foundations

Early training and socialization are critical for Australian Shepherds, known for their intelligence and energy. Here are the first steps in basic training:

- **Socialization**: Introduce your puppy to a variety of people, environments, and other animals. Positive experiences during this period are crucial for developing a well-adjusted adult dog.
- **Basic Commands**: Start with essential commands like "sit," "stay," "come," and "down." Use positive reinforcement methods, such as treats and praise, to encourage desired behaviors.
- **Leash Training**: Begin leash training early. Use a comfortable collar and leash, and practice short, positive walks. Teach your puppy to walk beside you without pulling.

- **Positive Reinforcement:** Reward-based training methods are effective for Australian Shepherds. Use treats, toys, and praise to reinforce good behavior and create a positive association with training sessions.

Chapter 2

Building a Strong Bond

Understanding Canine Communication

A strong bond with your Australian Shepherd begins with understanding how they communicate. Dogs use body language, vocalizations, and behavior to convey their feelings and intentions. Interpreting these signals accurately is essential for building a trusting relationship.

Reading Body Language

Australian Shepherds, like all dogs, communicate primarily through body language. Here are key signals to watch for and their meanings:

Tail Position and Movement:

- **Wagging Tail:** A wagging tail generally indicates happiness or excitement, but the speed and breadth of the wag can offer more clues. A slow wag can mean uncertainty, while a rapid, broad wag usually signifies joy.

- **Tail Down or Tucked**: A tail held down or tucked between the legs often signals fear, anxiety, or submission.
- **Tail High and Stiff**: A high, stiff tail can indicate alertness or assertiveness, and sometimes aggression.

Ears:

- **Ears Up and Forward**: Erect ears pointing forward typically show interest or alertness.
- **Ears Flattened or Back**: Ears held back against the head can indicate fear, submission, or discomfort.

Eyes:

- **Soft, Relaxed Eyes**: Soft, squinting eyes generally show relaxation and contentment.

- **Direct Stare**: A direct stare can be a sign of dominance or a challenge, especially if accompanied by stiff body language.
- **Whale Eye**: When a dog shows the whites of their eyes, it often signals fear or anxiety.

Mouth and Lips:

- **Relaxed Mouth**: A slightly open mouth, possibly with the tongue exposed, typically means the dog is relaxed.
- **Lip Licking or Yawning**: These behaviors can indicate stress or appeasement.
- **Bared Teeth**: Exposed teeth, especially with snarling or growling, are clear signs of aggression or fear.

Body Posture:

- **Relaxed Body**: A relaxed, loose body posture indicates the dog is comfortable and at ease.
- **Stiff Body**: A stiff, tense body can signal fear, aggression, or discomfort.

- **Cowering or Shrinking**: Cowering or making themselves appear smaller often signifies fear or submission.

The Importance of Socialization

Socialization is a critical aspect of raising a well-adjusted Australian Shepherd. It involves exposing your puppy to a variety of people, environments, sounds, and other animals in a positive manner. Here's why it's essential and how to do it effectively:

Benefits of Socialization:

- **Reduces Fear and Anxiety**: Proper socialization helps reduce fear and anxiety towards new experiences and environments.
- **Promotes Confidence**: A well-socialized dog is more confident and adaptable to different situations.
- **Prevents Behavioral Problems**: Early and positive exposure can prevent common

behavioral issues such as aggression, excessive barking, and fear-based reactions.

How to Socialize Your Australian Shepherd:

- **Start Early:** Begin socialization as early as possible, ideally during the puppy's critical socialization period (3-14 weeks of age).

- **Positive Experiences:** Ensure all new experiences are positive. Use treats, praise, and play to create positive associations.

- **Variety of Environments**: Expose your puppy to different environments, including parks, busy streets, car rides, and various types of flooring.

- **Different People and Animals:** Introduce your puppy to people of different ages, sizes, and appearances, as well as other dogs and animals.

- **Controlled Exposure:** Gradually increase the level of exposure. Start with quieter, controlled environments before moving to more stimulating settings.

Positive Reinforcement Training

Positive reinforcement is a powerful training method that strengthens the bond between you and your Australian Shepherd. It involves rewarding desirable behaviors to encourage their recurrence.

Basics of Reward-Based Training

The foundation of positive reinforcement training is simple: reward behaviors you want to see more often and ignore or redirect undesirable behaviors. Here's how to get started:

- **Identify Rewards:** Determine what motivates your dog. Common rewards include treats, toys, praise, and playtime.

High-value treats are particularly effective during training sessions.

- **Timing is Key**: Deliver the reward immediately after the desired behavior to create a clear association. The quicker the reward follows the behavior, the stronger the connection.

- **Consistency**: Be consistent with your commands and rewards. Everyone in the household should use the same commands and reward the same behaviors.

- **Start with Basic Commands**: Begin with simple commands like "sit," "stay," "come," and "down." These form the foundation for more advanced training.

- **Short Sessions**: Keep training sessions short and focused, typically around 5-10 minutes, to maintain your dog's interest and enthusiasm.

- **Gradual Progression**: Gradually increase the difficulty of commands and introduce distractions as your dog becomes more proficient.

Building Trust and Respect

Trust and respect are crucial components of a strong bond with your Australian Shepherd. Here's how to foster these qualities:

- **Be Patient**: Training takes time and patience. Avoid using punishment or negative reinforcement, as these can damage trust and create fear.
- **Consistent Routine:** Establish a consistent daily routine for feeding, exercise, training, and playtime. Consistency helps your dog feel secure and understand what to expect.
- **Positive Interactions**: Engage in positive interactions beyond training sessions. Spend quality time playing, walking, and simply being together.
- **Clear Communication:** Use clear, consistent commands and body language. Avoid mixed signals that can confuse your dog.

- **Respect Their Needs:** Understand and respect your dog's individual needs and preferences. Some Australian Shepherds may be more sensitive or independent than others.

Chapter 3

Basic Training Techniques

House Training

House training, also known as potty training, is one of the first and most crucial steps in ensuring your Australian Shepherd becomes a well-mannered member of your household. This process requires consistency, patience, and positive reinforcement.

Crate Training Method

Crate training is an effective house training technique that leverages a dog's natural instinct to keep their living area clean. Here's a detailed guide on how to crate train your Australian Shepherd:

Choosing the Right Crate:

- **Size**: Select a crate that is large enough for your dog to stand, turn around, and lie down comfortably but not so large that they can use one end as a bathroom.

- **Material**: Crates come in various materials, including wire, plastic, and fabric. Wire crates provide better ventilation and visibility, which can help your dog feel less confined.

Introducing the Crate:

- **Positive Association**: Introduce the crate as a positive space. Place it in a busy area of your home where your dog can see family activities.
- **Comfort**: Make the crate comfortable with soft bedding and a favorite toy.
- **Open Door Policy:** Leave the door open initially and allow your dog to explore the crate at their own pace. Use treats to encourage them to enter and stay inside for short periods.

Training Steps:

- **Feeding**: Feed your dog meals inside the crate to build positive associations. Start with the door open and gradually close it for short periods while they eat.

- **Short Periods:** Gradually increase the time your dog spends in the crate with the door closed. Begin with a few minutes and extend the duration gradually.
- **Potty Breaks**: Take your dog outside for potty breaks immediately after they exit the crate. Use a consistent phrase like "Go potty" and reward them for successful elimination outside.
- **Nighttime**: Place the crate near your bed initially to provide comfort during the night. As your dog becomes more comfortable, you can gradually move the crate to a preferred location.

Key Tips:

- **Consistency**: Maintain a consistent schedule for feeding, potty breaks, and crate time.

- **Avoid Punishment**: Never use the crate as a punishment, as this can create negative associations.
- **Patience**: Be patient and understanding. Crate training can take several weeks, and each dog progresses at their own pace.

Establishing a Routine

A consistent daily routine is essential for successful house training. Here's how to establish and maintain an effective routine:

Feeding Schedule:

- **Regular Meals:** Feed your dog at the same times each day to regulate their digestive system and predict potty needs.
- **Portion Control:** Provide measured portions to avoid overfeeding and ensure regular potty breaks.

Potty Break Schedule:

- **Frequent Breaks:** Take your puppy outside frequently, especially after waking up, eating, drinking, playing, and before bedtime.

- **Consistent Location:** Use the same outdoor spot for potty breaks to help your dog associate the area with elimination.
- **Positive Reinforcement:** Praise and reward your dog immediately after they eliminate outside. Use treats, praise, or play to reinforce good behavior.

Supervision and Confinement:

- **Close Supervision:** Supervise your dog closely when they are not in the crate. Watch for signs they need to go potty, such as sniffing, circling, or whining.
- **Short Absences:** When you can't supervise, confine your dog to a small, puppy-proofed area with easy-to-clean floors.

Accident Management:

- **Clean Thoroughly:** Clean accidents promptly and thoroughly to remove any lingering odor that might attract your dog to the same spot.

- **Avoid Punishment**: Never punish your dog for accidents. Instead, interrupt them if caught in the act and take them outside immediately.

Basic Commands

Training your Australian Shepherd to respond to basic commands is fundamental for their safety and good behavior. Here's a comprehensive guide to teaching the commands "Sit," "Stay," "Come," and "Heel," along with incorporating hand signals.

Sit

Teaching "Sit" is often the first command and lays the foundation for other training.

Steps to Teach "Sit":

- **Get Attention**: Hold a treat close to your dog's nose.

- **Lure:** Slowly move your hand up, allowing your dog's head to follow the treat and causing their bottom to lower.
- **Command:** As soon as their bottom touches the floor, say "Sit" and give the treat.
- **Praise:** Offer verbal praise and additional petting to reinforce the behavior.

Practice:

- **Repetition:** Practice several times a day in short sessions.
- **Gradual Distance:** Gradually increase the distance between you and your dog while giving the command.

Stay

"Stay" helps your dog learn impulse control and is useful in various situations.

Steps to Teach "Stay":

- **Command "Sit":** Start with your dog in the "Sit" position.

- **Hand Signal:** Hold your palm out in front of you, facing your dog, and say "Stay."
- **Step Back:** Take a step back and immediately step forward if your dog stays put. Reward them with a treat.
- **Increase Duration:** Gradually increase the time you ask your dog to stay before giving the treat.
- **Increase Distance:** Increase the distance between you and your dog slowly.

Practice:

- **Distraction:** Practice in various environments with different levels of distractions.
- **Consistency:** Use the same hand signal and verbal command each time.

Come

"Come" is a crucial command for your dog's safety and recall.

- Leash Training: Start training with your dog on a leash in a quiet area.
- Command: Crouch down, open your arms, and enthusiastically say "Come."
- Reward: When your dog comes to you, reward them with treats and praise.
- Increase Distance: Gradually increase the distance and practice off-leash in a safe, enclosed area.

Practice:

- Random Recall: Call your dog randomly during play or at home to reinforce the command.
- Positive Reinforcement: Always reward your dog when they come to you, even if they were distracted or it took some time.

Heel

"Heel" teaches your dog to walk beside you without pulling on the leash.

- Start Position: Begin with your dog sitting at your left side.
- Treats and Commands: Hold a treat in your left hand at your dog's nose level and say "Heel."
- Walk Slowly: Take a step forward, encouraging your dog to stay close to you by keeping the treat at their nose level.
- Praise and Reward: After a few steps, stop, praise, and reward your dog if they stayed by your side.

Practice:

- Gradual Progression: Increase the distance you walk together gradually.
- Distractions: Practice in various environments with different distractions to ensure reliability.

Incorporating Hand Signals

Hand signals can be a useful addition to verbal commands, providing clear visual cues for your dog. Here's how to incorporate hand signals into basic training:

Sit:

- Hand Signal: Raise your hand, palm facing upward, from your side to above your dog's head.
- Consistency: Use the hand signal each time you give the verbal "Sit" command until your dog responds to the signal alone.

Stay:

- Hand Signal: Hold your palm out in front of you, as if telling someone to stop.
- Consistency: Pair this signal with the verbal "Stay" command until your dog understands the signal alone.

Come:

- Hand Signal: Extend your arm out to the side and then bring it to your chest.
- Consistency: Use this signal along with the verbal "Come" command until your dog responds to the signal alone.

Heel:

- Hand Signal: Pat your left leg while saying "Heel."
- Consistency: Continue using this signal with the verbal command until your dog associates the signal with the action.

By following these detailed steps and techniques, you'll establish a strong foundation for further training and ensure your Australian Shepherd becomes a well-behaved, responsive, and happy member of your family.

Chapter 4

Advanced Training Techniques

Obedience Training

Once your Australian Shepherd has mastered basic commands, it's time to move on to more advanced obedience training. Advanced training not only enhances your dog's skills but also strengthens your bond and ensures their safety.

Off-Leash Training

Training your dog to behave off-leash is a significant achievement, providing them with more freedom while ensuring they remain under control.

Prerequisites:

- Basic Commands Mastery: Ensure your dog reliably responds to basic commands such as "Sit," "Stay," and "Come."

- Safe Environment: Start training in a secure, enclosed area where your dog can't escape or get into danger.

Steps to Off-Leash Training:

- Long Leash Transition:

Use a long training leash (15-30 feet) to give your dog more freedom while maintaining control. Practice basic commands and recall using the long leash. Gradually increase the distance between you and your dog.

- Reliable Recall:

Recall is crucial for off-leash training. Practice the "Come" command frequently, rewarding your dog every time they return to you.
Use high-value treats or toys to make returning to you the most rewarding option.

- Increase Distance and Distraction:

Gradually increase the distance and introduce distractions, such as other dogs or people, to test your dog's responsiveness.

Practice in different environments to ensure your dog can generalize the behavior.

- Off-Leash in Enclosed Area:

Once your dog consistently responds to commands on a long leash, try off-leash training in a safe, enclosed area.

Continue practicing recall and basic commands, rewarding your dog for compliance.

- Progress to Open Spaces:

When confident in an enclosed area, move to larger open spaces. Ensure the area is safe and free from potential hazards.

Maintain a high level of vigilance, especially in the beginning stages of off-leash training in open areas.

Key Tips:
- Stay Calm: Always remain calm and avoid chasing your dog if they run away. This can turn into a game for them.

- Regular Practice: Regularly practice off-leash commands to reinforce training.
- Safety First: Ensure your dog has proper identification and consider using a GPS tracker for added safety.

Reliable Recall

Reliable recall is essential for off-leash training and overall obedience. Here's an in-depth guide to achieving a reliable recall:

Foundational Steps:

- Establish a Recall Word:

Choose a specific word or phrase, such as "Come," "Here," or "Come here."
Ensure all family members use the same recall word consistently.

- Start Indoors:

Begin training in a distraction-free indoor environment.

Use treats or toys to encourage your dog to come to you. Crouch down, open your arms, and use your recall word enthusiastically.

- Use High-Value Rewards:

Use your dog's favorite treats or toys to make returning to you the most rewarding option.
Vary the rewards to keep your dog excited and motivated.

Advanced Recall Training:

- Introduce Distance:

Gradually increase the distance between you and your dog during recall training.
Use a long leash initially to ensure control while increasing distance.

- Add Distractions:

Introduce mild distractions and gradually increase their intensity.
Practice recall in different environments to help your dog generalize the command.

Proofing Recall:

Proofing involves testing your dog's recall in various real-life situations, such as around other dogs, people, or wildlife.
Reward heavily for successful recalls under challenging conditions.

Emergency Recall:

- Special Recall Word:

Choose a different word for emergency recall, such as "Emergency" or "Now."
Train this word separately, using the highest value rewards.

- High Stakes:

Use this recall word only in emergency situations or high-stakes training to maintain its significance.

Maintaining Recall:

- Regular Practice: Continue practicing recall regularly, even after your dog responds reliably.

- Positive Reinforcement: Always reward your dog for coming to you, even if it takes longer than desired.
- Games and Play: Incorporate recall into games and playtime to keep it fun and engaging.

Agility and Trick Training

Agility and trick training are excellent ways to keep your Australian Shepherd mentally and physically stimulated. These activities provide an outlet for their energy and intelligence.

Introduction to Agility

Agility training involves navigating a series of obstacles, such as jumps, tunnels, and weave poles. It's a fun, competitive sport that enhances your dog's coordination and obedience.

Benefits of Agility Training:

- Physical Exercise: Provides an excellent physical workout, helping to keep your dog fit and healthy.

- Mental Stimulation: Challenges your dog's mind, reducing boredom and associated behavioral problems.
- Bonding: Strengthens the bond between you and your dog through teamwork and communication.

Getting Started:

Basic Equipment:

- Jumps: Start with low jumps and gradually increase the height as your dog becomes more confident.
- Tunnels: Use short, straight tunnels initially. Gradually increase the length and introduce curved tunnels.
- Weave Poles: Begin with a few poles and increase the number as your dog's skills improve.

Foundation Training:

- Focus on Basics: Ensure your dog has mastered basic obedience commands.

- Introduce Obstacles Slowly: Introduce one obstacle at a time, using treats and praise to encourage your dog.

Training Techniques:

- Luring: Use a treat or toy to guide your dog through each obstacle.
- Shaping: Reward your dog for small steps towards completing an obstacle. Gradually raise the criteria for rewards.
- Targeting: Use a target stick or your hand to guide your dog through the course.

Building Courses:

- Simple Courses: Start with simple courses of 2-3 obstacles. Gradually add more obstacles as your dog gains confidence.
- Sequencing: Teach your dog to navigate multiple obstacles in sequence. Use verbal cues and hand signals to guide them.

Practice and Patience:
- Regular Practice: Practice regularly to build your dog's skills and confidence.

- Positive Reinforcement: Always use positive reinforcement. Avoid forcing your dog or showing frustration.

Fun Tricks to Stimulate Your Dog

Trick training is a fun way to engage your Australian Shepherd's mind and showcase their intelligence. Here are some enjoyable tricks to teach your dog:

Shake Hands:

Steps:
1. Have your dog sit.
2. Hold a treat in your hand and let your dog sniff it.
3. Close your hand around the treat and lift your dog's paw with your other hand, saying "Shake."
4. Reward your dog immediately.

Practice: Repeat several times until your dog lifts their paw on their own.

Roll Over:

Steps:

1. Have your dog lie down.
2. Hold a treat near their nose and slowly move it towards their shoulder, encouraging them to roll onto their side.
3. Continue moving the treat in a circular motion, encouraging your dog to complete the roll.
4. Say "Roll over" and reward your dog once they complete the trick.

Practice: Break the trick into smaller steps if needed, rewarding your dog for partial rolls initially.

Play Dead:

Steps:

1. Have your dog lie down.
2. Hold a treat near their nose and slowly move it towards their shoulder, encouraging them to roll onto their side.
3. Say "Bang" or "Play dead" and reward your dog for staying still.

Practice: Gradually increase the duration your dog stays in the "dead" position before rewarding.

Spin:

Steps:

1. Hold a treat close to your dog's nose.
2. Move the treat in a circular motion, encouraging your dog to follow it.
3. Say "Spin" as your dog completes the circle and reward them.

Practice: Gradually reduce the use of the treat as your dog learns the command.

Fetch:

Steps:

1. Choose a toy your dog likes.
2. Throw the toy a short distance.
3. Encourage your dog to retrieve it using excited tones and gestures.
4. Say "Fetch" and reward your dog when they bring the toy back.

Practice: Gradually increase the distance of the throw and use different toys.

Tips for Trick Training:

- Short Sessions: Keep training sessions short and fun to maintain your dog's interest.
- Positive Reinforcement: Use treats, praise, and play to reward your dog.
- Consistency: Use the same commands and hand signals each time.
- Patience: Be patient and break tricks into smaller steps if needed.

By progressing from basic to advanced training techniques, including obedience, off-leash, agility, and trick training, you'll ensure your Australian Shepherd remains mentally and physically stimulated. This will not only enhance their skills but also strengthen the bond between you and your dog, resulting in a happy, well-rounded companion.

Chapter 5

Socialization and Behavior

Importance of Early Socialization

Early socialization is critical for Australian Shepherds. It involves exposing your puppy to a variety of experiences, environments, people, and animals in a positive manner. This helps them develop into well-adjusted, confident adults and reduces the risk of behavioral issues.

Why Early Socialization is Important:

- Prevents Fearfulness: Puppies that aren't exposed to new experiences early on may become fearful of new situations later in life.
- Encourages Adaptability: Early socialization helps puppies adapt to new environments and changes in their routine.

- Promotes Positive Behavior: Well-socialized dogs are more likely to exhibit friendly and non-aggressive behaviors.
- Reduces Anxiety: Exposure to different stimuli helps puppies develop coping mechanisms for stress and anxiety.

Key Socialization Period:

Critical Window: The most crucial period for socialization is between 3 and 14 weeks of age. During this time, puppies are more open to new experiences and less likely to develop fear-based reactions.

Introducing New People and Pets

Introducing your Australian Shepherd to new people and pets is a significant part of their socialization process. Positive interactions with a variety of individuals and animals will help your dog develop good social skills and reduce the likelihood of fear or aggression.

Steps for Introducing New People:
- Controlled Environment:

Start introductions in a calm, controlled environment where your dog feels safe.

Keep initial interactions short and positive.

- Positive Associations:

Use treats and praise to create positive associations with new people.

Allow your dog to approach the new person at their own pace.

- Calm Behavior:

Encourage calm behavior from both your dog and the new person. Avoid loud noises or sudden movements.

Teach the new person to offer a closed hand for the dog to sniff before attempting to pet.

- Gradual Increase:

Gradually increase the number of people your dog meets. Start with one or two individuals and slowly introduce larger groups.

Include people of different ages, genders, and appearances to broaden your dog's experiences.

Steps for Introducing New Pets:
- Neutral Territory:

Introduce new pets in a neutral location to prevent territorial behavior.

Choose a quiet, outdoor space where both animals can feel comfortable.

- Leashed Introductions:

Keep both pets on a leash during the initial meeting to maintain control.

Allow them to sniff and investigate each other while keeping the leashes loose.

- Positive Reinforcement:

Use treats and praise to reward calm and friendly behavior.

Interrupt any signs of aggression or excessive excitement with a gentle distraction, like a toy or treat.

- **Supervised Interactions:**

Gradually increase the duration of interactions while closely supervising.

Monitor body language to ensure both animals are comfortable and relaxed.

- **Separate Spaces:**

Provide separate spaces for each pet initially, allowing them to get used to each other's presence gradually.

Use baby gates or crates to create safe zones where each pet can retreat if needed.

Positive Experiences in Different Environments

Exposing your Australian Shepherd to a variety of environments is crucial for their socialization. This helps them become well-rounded and adaptable, reducing the likelihood of fear or anxiety in new situations.

Steps for Introducing New Environments:

- Start Small:

Begin with familiar, low-stress environments, such as your backyard or a quiet park.

Gradually introduce new settings, like busy streets, shopping centers, or pet-friendly stores.

- Short Outings:

Keep initial outings short to prevent overwhelming your dog.

Gradually increase the duration as your dog becomes more comfortable.

- Positive Reinforcement:

Use treats, toys, and praise to reward your dog for calm behavior in new environments.

Create positive associations with each new place you visit.

- Varied Experiences:

Expose your dog to different surfaces, such as grass, gravel, sand, and pavement.

Include different types of weather, like rain or wind, to broaden their experiences.

- Controlled Exposure:

Introduce new sounds and sights gradually, such as traffic, construction noises, or crowded places.

Use distance to manage your dog's comfort level, gradually decreasing the distance as they become more confident.

Managing Common Behavioral Issues

Australian Shepherds are intelligent, energetic dogs that can develop behavioral issues if not properly trained and stimulated. Understanding and addressing these issues early can prevent them from becoming problematic.

Addressing Barking, Chewing, and Digging
Barking:

- Identify the Cause:

Determine the reason for the barking: boredom, anxiety, attention-seeking, or alerting.
Address the root cause rather than just the symptom.

- Training Commands:

Teach the "Quiet" command. Use a treat to reward silence and gradually increase the duration.
Use a consistent command and reward system to reinforce desired behavior.

- Reduce Triggers:

Minimize exposure to triggers that cause barking, such as closing blinds to block visual stimuli.
Provide background noise, like a TV or white noise machine, to mask outside sounds.

- Exercise and Mental Stimulation:

Ensure your dog gets plenty of physical exercise and mental stimulation to prevent boredom-induced barking.

Use puzzle toys, training sessions, and interactive play to keep your dog engaged.

Chewing:

- Provide Appropriate Chews:

Offer a variety of chew toys to satisfy your dog's natural chewing instincts.
Rotate toys to keep your dog interested and prevent boredom.

- Manage the Environment:

Puppy-proof your home by removing or securing items your dog might chew on.
Use baby gates or crates to limit access to off-limits areas.

- Training Redirection:

Interrupt inappropriate chewing with a gentle "No" or "Leave it" command.
Redirect your dog to an appropriate chew toy and reward them for using it.

- Exercise and Mental Stimulation:

Ensure your dog gets enough physical exercise and mental enrichment to reduce boredom and anxiety.

Use chew toys that also provide mental stimulation, like treat-dispensing toys or puzzle feeders.

Digging:

- Identify the Cause:

Determine why your dog is digging: boredom, hunting instincts, cooling off, or hiding objects.

Address the underlying cause to reduce the behavior.

- Designated Digging Area:

Create a designated digging area in your yard where your dog is allowed to dig.

Bury toys or treats in the designated area to encourage digging there.

- Supervise and Redirect:

Supervise your dog when outside and redirect them to the designated digging area if they start digging elsewhere.

Use positive reinforcement to reward digging in the appropriate area.

- Exercise and Mental Stimulation:

Provide ample physical exercise and mental stimulation to prevent boredom-induced digging.

Use interactive toys, training sessions, and play to keep your dog engaged.

Handling Separation Anxiety

Separation anxiety is a common issue in dogs, including Australian Shepherds. It occurs when a dog becomes distressed when left alone. Addressing this issue early is crucial for your dog's well-being.

Signs of Separation Anxiety:

1. Excessive barking, howling, or whining when left alone

2. Destructive behavior, such as chewing furniture or digging at doors and windows
3. Pacing, panting, or drooling
4. Attempting to escape from confinement
5. Steps to Address Separation Anxiety:

Gradual Desensitization:

1. Gradually accustom your dog to being alone. Start with short absences and gradually increase the duration.
2. Use a consistent routine for departures and arrivals to reduce anxiety.

Positive Associations:

- Create positive associations with being alone by providing special toys or treats that your dog only gets when you leave.
- Use puzzle feeders or treat-dispensing toys to keep your dog occupied.

Practice Calm Departures and Arrivals:

- Avoid making a big fuss when leaving or returning home. Keep your departures and arrivals calm and low-key.
- Ignore your dog for a few minutes before you leave and after you return to reduce excitement and anxiety.

Provide a Safe Space:
- Create a comfortable, safe space for your dog, such as a crate or a designated room.
- Ensure the area has familiar bedding, toys, and a water source.

Exercise and Mental Stimulation:
- Provide ample physical exercise and mental stimulation before leaving to tire your dog out and reduce anxiety.
- Use training sessions, interactive toys, and play to keep your dog engaged.

Consider Professional Help:

- If your dog's separation anxiety is severe, consider seeking help from a professional dog trainer or behaviorist.
- In some cases, your veterinarian may recommend medication to help manage anxiety.

By understanding the importance of early socialization, properly introducing new people and pets, providing positive experiences in different environments, and effectively managing common behavioral issues, you can ensure your Australian Shepherd develops into a well-adjusted, confident, and happy companion.

Chapter 6

Health and Nutrition

Diet and Nutrition

Proper diet and nutrition are essential for the overall health and well-being of your Australian Shepherd. A balanced diet ensures your dog receives the necessary nutrients to maintain a healthy weight, support growth, and promote a long, active life.

Choosing the Right Food

Selecting the right food for your Australian Shepherd involves considering factors such as age, size, activity level, and any specific health concerns. Here are the key considerations:

Life Stage:
- Puppy: Puppies require food formulated to support growth and development. Look for

puppy-specific formulas rich in protein, fats, and essential vitamins.

- Adult: Adult dogs need a balanced diet that maintains their energy levels and overall health. Choose high-quality adult dog food with balanced nutrients.
- Senior: Senior dogs may require food with fewer calories but higher fiber to manage weight and support digestive health. Senior formulas often include joint support supplements like glucosamine and chondroitin.

Quality Ingredients:
- Opt for dog food with high-quality, natural ingredients. Avoid foods with artificial preservatives, colors, and flavors.
- Look for meat or fish as the primary ingredient, indicating a high protein content.

- Choose foods with whole grains, fruits, and vegetables for added fiber, vitamins, and minerals.

Specific Needs:

- If your dog has specific health issues, such as allergies or digestive problems, consider special formulas designed to address these needs.
- Consult your veterinarian to determine if your dog requires a prescription diet or specific supplements.

Types of Dog Food:

- Dry Kibble: Convenient and long-lasting, dry kibble helps keep teeth clean and supports oral health.
- Wet/Canned Food: Higher in moisture, wet food is often more palatable and can be beneficial for dogs with dental issues or those needing extra hydration.
- Raw/Fresh Food: Raw or fresh diets can provide high-quality nutrition but require

careful handling and preparation to avoid contamination.

Understanding Nutritional Needs

To ensure your Australian Shepherd's diet meets their nutritional needs, it's important to understand the key nutrients required:

- Protein:

Essential for muscle development and maintenance, protein should be the primary component of your dog's diet.
Sources include meat, fish, poultry, and eggs.

- Fats:

Fats provide energy and support healthy skin and coat. Look for sources like fish oil, chicken fat, and flaxseed.
Omega-3 and Omega-6 fatty acids are particularly important for coat health and reducing inflammation.

- Carbohydrates:

Carbohydrates provide energy and fiber. Whole grains, vegetables, and fruits are good sources. Fiber aids in digestion and helps maintain a healthy weight.

- Vitamins and Minerals:

Vitamins (A, D, E, K, and B-complex) and minerals (calcium, phosphorus, potassium, and zinc) are crucial for overall health.

Ensure your dog's food includes a balanced blend of these nutrients.

- Water:

Always provide fresh, clean water. Proper hydration is vital for digestion, circulation, and temperature regulation.

Regular Health Check-Ups

Regular health check-ups are vital for preventing and detecting health issues early. Routine veterinary visits allow for timely vaccinations, preventive care, and monitoring of your dog's overall health.

Vaccinations and Preventive Care

Core Vaccinations:

Core vaccines protect against common, serious diseases. These typically include:

- Distemper: Protects against a highly contagious viral disease affecting the respiratory, gastrointestinal, and nervous systems.
- Parvovirus: Prevents a potentially fatal virus that causes severe gastrointestinal symptoms.
- Canine Hepatitis: Protects against infectious canine hepatitis, affecting the liver and other organs.
- Rabies: Required by law in many areas, this vaccine protects against a deadly virus transmissible to humans.

Non-Core Vaccinations:

Depending on your dog's lifestyle and environment, additional vaccines may be recommended:

- Bordetella (Kennel Cough): Recommended for dogs frequently in contact with other dogs, such as in boarding or daycare settings.
- Leptospirosis: Protects against a bacterial infection that can be transmitted through water or soil contaminated with urine from infected animals.
- Lyme Disease: Recommended for dogs in areas where Lyme disease is prevalent.

Parasite Prevention:

- Regular treatments for fleas, ticks, and heartworms are essential. Discuss the best preventive measures with your veterinarian.
- Use flea and tick preventatives year-round, and administer monthly heartworm medication.

Dental Care:
- Regular dental check-ups and cleanings help prevent periodontal disease.
- Brush your dog's teeth regularly and provide dental chews to maintain oral health.

Routine Blood Work and Screenings:
- Annual blood work helps detect underlying health issues, such as kidney or liver disease, early.
- Screenings for conditions like hip dysplasia or hereditary diseases may be recommended, especially as your dog ages.

Identifying Common Health Issues

Being aware of common health issues in Australian Shepherds and recognizing early signs can lead to prompt treatment and better outcomes.

Hip Dysplasia:

- Signs: Lameness, difficulty rising, reluctance to jump or climb stairs, and decreased activity.
- Management: Maintain a healthy weight, provide joint supplements, and consider physical therapy or surgery in severe cases.

Elbow Dysplasia:

- Signs: Lameness, swelling, and pain in the elbows.
- Management: Weight management, joint supplements, anti-inflammatory medications, and surgery if necessary.

Progressive Retinal Atrophy (PRA):

- Signs: Night blindness, dilated pupils, and progressive vision loss.
- Management: No cure exists, but regular veterinary check-ups can help monitor the condition. Genetic testing before breeding can prevent PRA.

Epilepsy:

- Signs: Seizures of varying intensity, from mild to severe.
- Management: Anti-seizure medications and regular veterinary monitoring.

Allergies:

- Signs: Itching, skin infections, ear infections, and gastrointestinal issues.
- Management: Identify and avoid allergens, use hypoallergenic diets, and consider medications to manage symptoms.

Hypothyroidism:

- Signs: Weight gain, lethargy, hair loss, and skin issues.
- Management: Lifelong thyroid hormone replacement therapy.

Collie Eye Anomaly (CEA):

- Signs: Varies from mild to severe vision impairment.

- Management: Regular eye exams and genetic testing before breeding.

Deafness:

- Signs: Lack of response to sounds, difficulty waking, and increased startle response.
- Management: Training and communication techniques tailored to deaf dogs, such as hand signals and vibration collars.

By understanding the dietary and nutritional needs of your Australian Shepherd, providing regular health check-ups, vaccinations, preventive care, and being aware of common health issues, you can ensure your dog leads a healthy, happy, and active life.

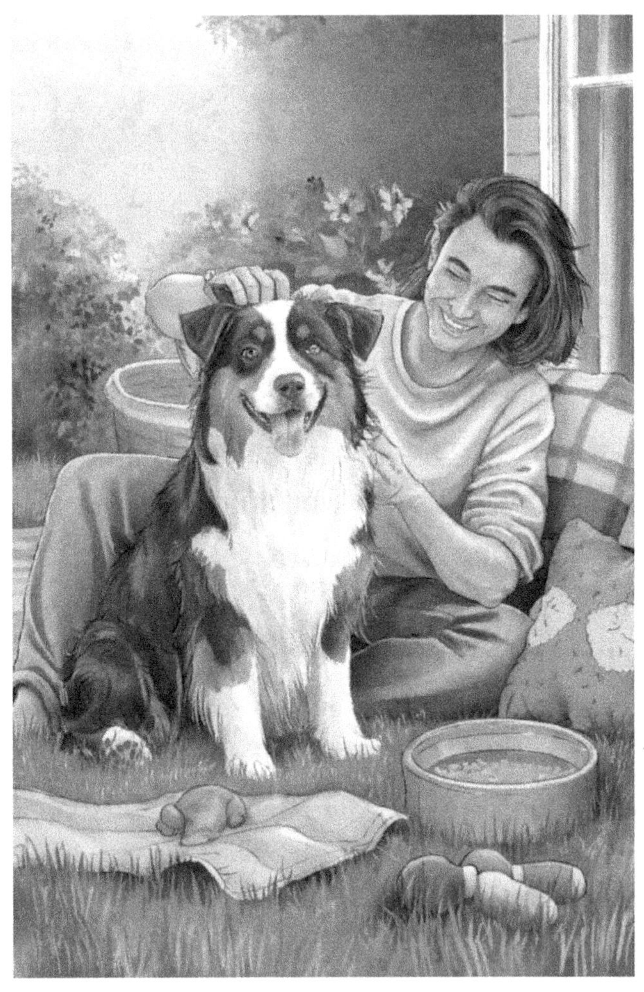

Chapter 7

Grooming and Care

Coat Care and Grooming Techniques

Proper grooming is essential for maintaining your Australian Shepherd's health and appearance. Their double coat requires regular maintenance to prevent matting, control shedding, and keep their skin healthy.

Brushing and Bathing

Brushing:

Regular brushing is crucial for keeping your Australian Shepherd's coat healthy and free of tangles and mats. Here's how to do it effectively:

Frequency:

- Daily Brushing: Ideally, brush your Australian Shepherd daily to remove loose hair and prevent tangles.
- Weekly Brushing: At a minimum, aim for thorough brushing at least twice a week.

Tools:

- Slicker Brush: Effective for removing loose hair and detangling.
- Undercoat Rake: Useful for reaching the dense undercoat and reducing shedding.
- Comb: Helps in detailing and removing remaining tangles or mats.

Technique:

- Start with a Slicker Brush: Begin by gently brushing your dog's coat with a slicker brush, focusing on one section at a time.
- Use the Undercoat Rake: Follow up with an undercoat rake to remove loose hair from the dense undercoat.

- Comb for Details: Finish by combing through the coat to catch any remaining tangles or mats.

Mat Removal:

- Identify Mats: Check for mats, especially behind the ears, under the legs, and along the tail.
- Detangle Gently: Use a detangling spray if needed and gently work out mats with your fingers or a comb. Be patient and avoid pulling hard, which can hurt your dog.

Bathing:

Bathing is important but should not be too frequent to avoid stripping natural oils from your dog's coat.

Frequency:

- Regular Baths: Bathe your Australian Shepherd every 6-8 weeks or as needed, depending on their activity level and dirt accumulation.

Products:

- Dog-Specific Shampoo: Use a high-quality, dog-specific shampoo. Avoid human shampoos, which can be too harsh for your dog's skin.
- Conditioner: A dog conditioner can help keep the coat soft and manageable, especially if your dog's coat is prone to dryness or tangling.

Bathing Process:

- Prepare the Area: Use a non-slip mat in the bathtub or grooming area to prevent slipping.
- Wet Thoroughly: Wet your dog's coat thoroughly with lukewarm water.
- Apply Shampoo: Apply shampoo and lather, focusing on one section at a time. Be gentle around the face and avoid getting shampoo in the eyes and ears.

- Rinse Well: Rinse thoroughly to remove all shampoo residues, which can cause skin irritation if left in the coat.
- Apply Conditioner: If using a conditioner, apply it and let it sit for a few minutes before rinsing.
- Drying: Use a towel to remove excess water. Follow up with a blow dryer on a low, cool setting to avoid overheating the skin. Brush the coat while drying to prevent tangles.

Dealing with Shedding

Australian Shepherds are moderate to heavy shedders, particularly during seasonal changes. Managing shedding helps keep your home clean and reduces the risk of matting.

Regular Brushing:
- Daily brushing during shedding seasons (spring and fall) helps control loose hair.
- Use an undercoat rake to reach and remove the dense undercoat effectively.

Deshedding Tools:

- Furminator: A deshedding tool like the Furminator can be very effective in reducing loose hair.
- Slicker Brush and Undercoat Rake: Combined use of these tools helps manage both topcoat and undercoat shedding.

Diet and Health:

- Balanced Diet: Ensure your dog is on a balanced diet rich in Omega-3 and Omega-6 fatty acids, which promote healthy skin and coat.
- Hydration: Proper hydration supports skin health and reduces excessive shedding.

Regular Baths:

- Regular baths help remove loose hair and keep the coat clean, reducing the amount of shedding.

Dental and Ear Care

Maintaining your Australian Shepherd's oral hygiene and ear cleanliness is crucial for their overall health. Regular care prevents dental diseases and ear infections.

Maintaining Oral Hygiene

Dental care is essential for preventing plaque buildup, gum disease, and bad breath.

Brushing Teeth:

- Frequency: Brush your dog's teeth daily or at least 3-4 times a week.
- Toothpaste: Use a dog-specific toothpaste. Never use human toothpaste, which can be harmful if swallowed.
- Toothbrush: A soft-bristled dog toothbrush or finger brush works well.

Brushing Technique:

- Introduce Gradually: Start by letting your dog get used to the taste of the toothpaste. Gradually introduce the toothbrush.

- Lift the Lip: Gently lift your dog's lip and brush in small, circular motions, focusing on the gum line.
- Be Patient: Take your time and make the experience positive with praise and treats.

Dental Chews and Toys:

- Chew Toys: Provide dental chew toys that help clean teeth as your dog chews.
- Dental Treats: Dental treats can help reduce plaque and tartar buildup.

Professional Cleanings:

- Schedule regular professional dental cleanings with your veterinarian. These cleanings allow for thorough plaque and tartar removal.

Cleaning Ears Safely

Regular ear cleaning helps prevent infections, especially in breeds prone to ear problems like the Australian Shepherd.

Frequency:

- Check Weekly: Check your dog's ears weekly for signs of dirt, wax buildup, or infection.
- Clean Monthly: Clean the ears monthly or as needed, depending on the accumulation of wax and debris.

Cleaning Products:

- Ear Cleaner: Use a veterinarian-recommended ear cleaner.
- Cotton Balls: Use cotton balls or pads for cleaning. Avoid cotton swabs, which can push debris further into the ear canal.

Cleaning Process:

- Inspect: Look inside your dog's ears for redness, swelling, or unusual discharge. A healthy ear should be pink and clean with no strong odor.

- Apply Cleaner: Apply the ear cleaner according to the product instructions. Fill the ear canal and gently massage the base of the ear to loosen debris.
- Wipe Out: Use a cotton ball or pad to wipe out the loosened debris. Repeat if necessary, but avoid inserting anything deep into the ear canal.
- Dry Ears: Ensure the ears are dry after cleaning to prevent moisture buildup, which can lead to infections.

Monitor for Infections:

- Signs of Infection: Be aware of signs such as redness, swelling, foul odor, excessive scratching, or head shaking.
- Consult Your Vet: If you notice any signs of infection, consult your veterinarian for appropriate treatment.

Conclusion

Grooming and care are essential aspects of maintaining the health and well-being of your Australian Shepherd. Regular brushing and bathing keep their coat healthy and free from mats and tangles, while dealing with shedding helps manage loose hair. Dental and ear care prevent common health issues such as periodontal disease and ear infections. By incorporating these grooming routines into your dog's care regimen, you ensure they remain comfortable, healthy, and happy throughout their life.

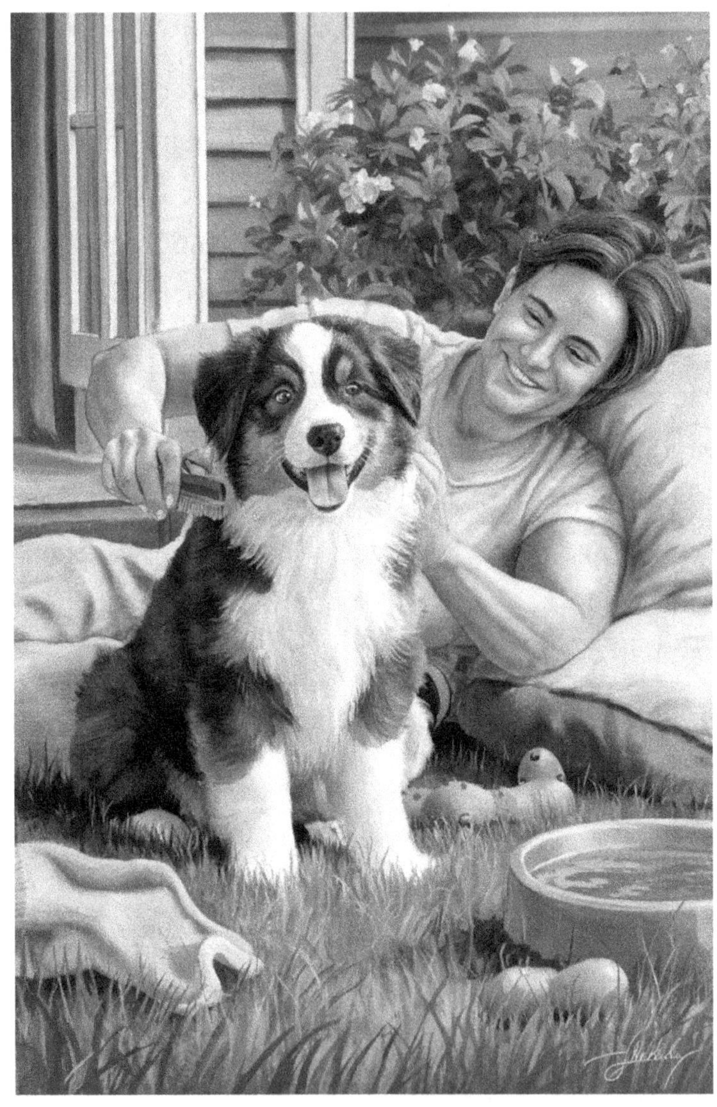

Chapter 8

Exercise and Mental Stimulation

Daily Exercise Needs

Australian Shepherds are an active and energetic breed that requires substantial daily exercise to maintain their physical and mental health. Proper exercise helps prevent behavioral issues, supports overall well-being, and strengthens the bond between you and your dog.

Walks, Runs, and Playtime

Walks:

- Daily Walks: Aim for at least one to two hours of walking per day. Break this into two sessions if possible – one in the morning and one in the evening.
- Vary the Route: Change the walking routes frequently to provide new sights, smells,

and experiences, which help keep your dog mentally stimulated.

- Leash Training: Ensure your dog is well-trained on a leash to make walks enjoyable for both of you. Teach them to walk beside you without pulling.

Runs:

- High Energy Needs: Australian Shepherds have high energy levels and can benefit greatly from regular running sessions.
- Jogging Partner: They make excellent jogging partners. Start with shorter distances and gradually increase as your dog builds stamina.
- Safety First: Always run in safe areas away from heavy traffic, and be mindful of extreme weather conditions that might be too hot or cold for your dog.

Playtime:

- Fetch: Playing fetch is an excellent way to exercise your Australian Shepherd. Use balls, frisbees, or other toys that your dog enjoys.

- Tug-of-War: This game provides both physical and mental exercise. Ensure you use a sturdy toy and teach your dog the "drop it" command to maintain control.
- Dog Parks: Socializing and playing with other dogs at a dog park can provide great exercise and help with socialization skills. Supervise interactions to ensure they are positive and safe.

Importance of Consistent Activity

Consistent physical activity is crucial for the health and happiness of Australian Shepherds. Inconsistent or insufficient exercise can lead to various issues:

- Behavioral Problems:

Lack of exercise can result in destructive behaviors such as chewing, digging, and excessive barking. These behaviors are often signs of boredom or pent-up energy.

- Weight Management:

Regular exercise helps maintain a healthy weight, reducing the risk of obesity-related health problems such as diabetes, heart disease, and joint issues.

- Mental Health:

Physical activity also supports mental health. It reduces stress and anxiety and helps prevent depression by providing mental stimulation and engagement.

- Bonding:

Exercise time is an excellent opportunity to strengthen the bond between you and your dog. Interactive play and training during exercise sessions build trust and communication.

Mental Enrichment

In addition to physical exercise, mental enrichment is vital for the well-being of Australian Shepherds. These intelligent dogs thrive on mental challenges and problem-solving activities.

Puzzle Toys and Interactive Games

Puzzle Toys:
- Types of Puzzle Toys: Invest in a variety of puzzle toys that require your dog to solve problems to receive treats or toys. Examples include treat-dispensing balls, puzzle boards, and interactive feeders.
- Difficulty Levels: Start with simpler puzzles and gradually introduce more complex ones as your dog becomes more proficient.
- Benefits: Puzzle toys provide mental stimulation, reduce boredom, and can be particularly helpful for dogs with separation anxiety.

Interactive Games:
- Hide and Seek: Hide treats or toys around the house or yard and encourage your dog

to find them. This game stimulates their natural hunting instincts and keeps them engaged.

- Treasure Hunt: Create a treasure hunt by hiding treats or toys under cups or in boxes. Teach your dog to find the hidden items, enhancing their problem-solving skills.
- Training Games: Incorporate training into playtime. Use games that require your dog to follow commands or perform tricks, such as "find it," "hide and seek," or agility exercises.

Training Exercises for Mental Sharpness

Obedience Training:
- Advanced Commands: Once your dog has mastered basic commands like sit, stay, come, and heel, introduce more advanced commands and tricks. This keeps their mind sharp and engaged.

- Regular Sessions: Hold regular training sessions to reinforce learned commands and introduce new ones. Keep sessions short (10-15 minutes) and fun to maintain interest.

Agility Training:

- Agility Courses: Set up a basic agility course in your yard or join an agility class. Activities such as jumping over hurdles, weaving through poles, and navigating tunnels provide both physical and mental stimulation.
- Benefits: Agility training improves coordination, enhances obedience, and provides an outlet for your dog's energy.

Scent Work:

- Nose Work: Engage your dog's powerful sense of smell with scent work activities. Hide treats or toys and encourage your dog to use their nose to find them.

- Scent Training: Enroll in a nose work class or create scent trails in your home or yard. This type of training is mentally enriching and taps into your dog's natural instincts.

Interactive Play:

- Tug Games: Play tug-of-war with a rope toy, incorporating commands like "take it," "drop it," and "leave it" to make the game mentally engaging.
- Fetch with Commands: When playing fetch, add commands such as "sit," "stay," and "wait" before allowing your dog to retrieve the toy. This reinforces obedience and provides mental stimulation.

Daily Challenges:

- Routine Variations: Change up your daily routines to keep things interesting for your dog. Introduce new walking routes, different training exercises, and varied play activities.

- Learning New Tricks: Continuously teach your dog new tricks and commands. This not only keeps their mind sharp but also strengthens your bond.

Conclusion

Proper exercise and mental stimulation are essential components of a healthy and happy life for Australian Shepherds. By providing consistent physical activity through walks, runs, and playtime, you help maintain their physical health and prevent behavioral issues. Mental enrichment through puzzle toys, interactive games, and training exercises keeps their intelligent minds engaged and sharp. Balancing both physical and mental activities ensures your Australian Shepherd thrives and enjoys a fulfilling life with you.

Chapter 9

Preparing for Different Life Stages

Puppyhood to Adulthood

Australian Shepherds go through distinct life stages, each requiring specific care, training adjustments, and attention. Understanding how to cater to these changing needs ensures your dog remains healthy, happy, and well-behaved throughout their life.

Transitioning Training Techniques

Puppyhood (0-6 Months):

- Basic Training: Focus on basic obedience training, including commands such as sit, stay, come, and heel. Use positive reinforcement techniques to build trust and encourage learning.

- Socialization: Introduce your puppy to various environments, people, and other animals to promote healthy social behavior. Puppy classes can be very beneficial.
- House Training: Establish a consistent routine for potty training. Use crate training to assist with this process and to provide a safe space for your puppy.

Adolescence (6-18 Months):
- Increasing Difficulty: As your dog matures, increase the complexity of training exercises. Introduce advanced commands and tricks to keep their mind engaged.
- Consistency and Patience: Adolescence can be a challenging period with increased independence and testing of boundaries. Maintain consistent training routines and be patient.
- Physical Exercise: Increase the intensity and duration of physical activities to

match their growing energy levels. Incorporate activities like agility training, fetch, and running.

Adulthood (18 Months - 7 Years):
- Advanced Training: Continue to build on advanced obedience and introduce specialized training such as herding, agility, or nose work, depending on your dog's interests and abilities.
- Mental Stimulation: Ensure ongoing mental enrichment with puzzle toys, interactive games, and regular training sessions.
- Physical Maintenance: Maintain a regular exercise routine that includes both physical and mental challenges. Monitor their diet and weight to prevent obesity.

Transitioning Training Techniques:

- Adapt to Needs: As your dog transitions from puppyhood to adulthood, adjust training techniques to suit their developmental stage. Use age-appropriate challenges and maintain a balance between physical and mental stimulation.

- Reinforcement: Continuously reinforce previously learned behaviors and commands to prevent regression and to keep their skills sharp.

Adjusting Care as They Grow

Nutrition:

- Puppy Nutrition: Puppies require a diet rich in protein, fats, and essential nutrients to support growth and development. Feed them high-quality puppy food and adjust portions as they grow.
- Adult Nutrition: Transition to adult dog food at around 12-18 months. Choose a balanced diet suitable for their activity level and health needs.
- Regular Monitoring: Regularly monitor your dog's weight and adjust their diet accordingly. Consult your veterinarian for

dietary recommendations based on your dog's specific needs.

Health Check-Ups:

- Puppy Visits: Schedule regular veterinary visits during the first year for vaccinations, deworming, and general health checks.

- Annual Exams: Continue with annual veterinary exams throughout adulthood to monitor health, update vaccinations, and address any concerns.

- Senior Screenings: As your dog ages, increase the frequency of health check-ups to detect and manage age-related conditions early.

Grooming:

- Early Introduction: Introduce grooming routines early to get your puppy accustomed to brushing, bathing, and nail trimming.

- Consistent Grooming: Maintain regular grooming throughout your dog's life to keep their coat healthy and free of mats and tangles.

- Age-Appropriate Tools: Use grooming tools suitable for your dog's coat type and age. Older dogs may require gentler tools and more frequent grooming sessions to manage shedding and skin health.

Exercise and Mental Stimulation:

- Age-Appropriate Activities: Tailor exercise routines to your dog's age and energy levels. Puppies need shorter, more frequent play sessions, while adults can handle more intense activities.

- Mental Challenges: Continuously provide mental challenges suitable for your dog's developmental stage. Increase complexity as they grow to keep their mind sharp.

Senior Dog Care

As your Australian Shepherd enters their senior years, their needs will change. Providing appropriate care during this stage ensures they remain comfortable, healthy, and happy.

Health Considerations for Older Dogs

Regular Veterinary Care:
- Frequent Check-Ups: Schedule more frequent veterinary visits, ideally every six months, to monitor for age-related health issues.
- Blood Work and Screenings: Regular blood tests and screenings help detect conditions such as kidney disease, liver issues, diabetes, and thyroid problems early.
- Vaccinations and Preventive Care: Keep up with vaccinations, dental care, and parasite prevention. Discuss any changes in your dog's health with your veterinarian promptly.

Diet and Nutrition:

- Senior Dog Food: Transition to a senior-specific dog food that is lower in calories but higher in fiber and joint-supporting supplements like glucosamine and chondroitin.
- Weight Management: Monitor your dog's weight closely, as obesity can exacerbate joint problems and other health issues. Adjust portions and provide a balanced diet.
- Hydration: Ensure your dog has access to fresh water at all times. Senior dogs may need to drink more due to changes in kidney function or medication side effects.

Joint and Mobility Care:

- Joint Supplements: Provide joint supplements such as glucosamine and chondroitin to support joint health and mobility.

- Comfortable Bedding: Ensure your dog has a comfortable, supportive bed to help reduce pressure on their joints.
- Manage Arthritis: If your dog shows signs of arthritis, such as stiffness or reluctance to move, consult your veterinarian. Medications, physical therapy, and lifestyle adjustments can help manage pain and improve mobility.

Keeping Senior Dogs Active and Engaged

Gentle Exercise:

- Low-Impact Activities: Engage in low-impact exercises such as leisurely walks, gentle play, and swimming. Avoid high-impact activities that could stress their joints.
- Consistency: Maintain a regular exercise routine to keep your dog active and prevent muscle loss. Adjust the intensity

and duration based on their comfort and ability.

Mental Stimulation:

- Puzzle Toys: Continue to provide puzzle toys and interactive games that challenge your dog's mind and prevent cognitive decline.

- Training: Incorporate training exercises that are appropriate for your senior dog's physical capabilities. Teaching new tricks or reinforcing old ones keeps their mind sharp.

- Environmental Enrichment: Provide a stimulating environment with new smells, toys, and experiences. Rotate toys regularly to keep them interesting.

Social Interaction:

- Companionship: Ensure your senior dog gets plenty of social interaction with family members and other pets. Loneliness and isolation can lead to depression and anxiety.

- Gentle Playdates: Arrange gentle playdates with other friendly dogs, if your dog enjoys socializing. Monitor interactions to ensure they remain positive and stress-free.

Comfort and Routine:

- Consistent Routine: Maintain a consistent daily routine to provide a sense of security and stability. Sudden changes can cause stress and anxiety in older dogs.
- Comfort Measures: Make your home more senior-friendly by providing ramps or steps to help your dog access furniture, and keep their living area warm and draft-free.

Conclusion

Preparing for the different life stages of your Australian Shepherd involves adapting your care, training, and attention to their changing needs.

From puppyhood to adulthood and into their senior years, understanding and meeting these needs ensures your dog remains healthy, happy, and well-adjusted. By providing appropriate nutrition, regular health check-ups, consistent exercise, mental stimulation, and specialized senior care, you can enjoy a long, fulfilling life with your beloved Australian Shepherd.

Chapter 10

Traveling with Your Australian Shepherd

Traveling with your Australian Shepherd can be an enriching experience for both you and your pet. Whether you're planning a short car ride or an extended vacation, it's essential to ensure that your dog's safety, comfort, and well-being are prioritized. This chapter covers everything you need to know for successful and enjoyable travel with your Australian Shepherd, from car travel tips to vacationing together.

Car Travel Tips

Traveling by car is often the most convenient way to transport your Australian Shepherd. Proper preparation and adherence to safety precautions can make the journey pleasant for both you and your dog.

Safety Precautions

Secure Restraints:
- Dog Seat Belts and Harnesses: Use a specially designed dog seat belt or harness to secure your Australian Shepherd in the car. This prevents them from moving around and reduces the risk of injury in case of sudden stops or accidents.
- Crates and Carriers: For smaller dogs or long trips, a sturdy crate or carrier is an excellent option. Ensure the crate is well-ventilated, spacious enough for your dog to stand, turn around, and lie down comfortably, and securely fastened in the car.

Comfortable Environment:
- Temperature Control: Keep the car well-ventilated and maintain a comfortable temperature. Never leave your dog in a parked car, especially in extreme weather

conditions, as it can quickly become dangerously hot or cold.

- Regular Breaks: Schedule regular breaks every 2-3 hours to allow your dog to stretch, relieve themselves, and have some water. This helps prevent restlessness and discomfort during long trips.

Proper Positioning:

- Back Seat: Place your dog in the back seat of the car. The front seat can be dangerous due to airbags, which can cause serious injuries to dogs in case of deployment.
- Window Safety: Ensure the windows are not fully open to prevent your dog from attempting to jump out. Use window guards or keep the windows only slightly open for ventilation.

Reducing Travel Anxiety

Familiarization:

- Short Rides: Start by taking your dog on short car rides to help them get used to the motion and environment. Gradually increase the length of the trips as they become more comfortable.
- Positive Associations: Make car rides a positive experience by offering treats, praise, and toys during and after the ride. This helps your dog associate car travel with enjoyable activities.

Comfort Items:

- Favorite Toys and Blankets: Bring along your dog's favorite toys and blankets to provide comfort and a sense of familiarity during the trip.

Chapter 11

Building a Routine

Creating a consistent and balanced daily routine is essential for the well-being of your Australian Shepherd. A structured schedule provides your dog with a sense of security, helps manage their energy levels, and fosters good behavior. This chapter covers how to build an effective daily routine, the importance of consistency, and how to adjust to changes, such as moving to a new home or coping with life transitions.

Daily Schedules

A well-structured daily schedule for your Australian Shepherd should include time for feeding, exercise, training, play, grooming, and rest. Here's a comprehensive guide to creating a balanced routine:

Morning Routine

Wake-Up and Potty Break:
- Consistent Wake-Up Time: Establish a regular wake-up time to help your dog start the day with a sense of routine.
- Morning Potty Break: Take your dog outside for a potty break as soon as they wake up. This helps prevent accidents and sets a positive tone for the day.

Feeding:
- Breakfast: Feed your dog a balanced breakfast. Ensure the meal is nutritionally complete and appropriate for their age, weight, and activity level.
- Hydration: Provide fresh water and encourage your dog to drink.

Exercise:

- Morning Walk: Take your dog for a morning walk to burn off excess energy and stimulate their mind. Aim for at least 30-60 minutes of walking, incorporating some playtime if possible.
- Interactive Play: Engage in interactive play, such as fetch or tug-of-war, to further stimulate your dog both physically and mentally.

Training:

- Training Session: Incorporate a short training session to practice obedience commands and introduce new skills. Morning is an excellent time for training as your dog is alert and focused.

Midday Routine

Potty Break:

- Midday Potty Break: Take your dog outside for a potty break around midday to prevent accidents and provide a change of scenery.

Mental Stimulation:

- Puzzle Toys: Provide puzzle toys or interactive feeders to keep your dog mentally stimulated while you're busy or at work.
- Scent Work: Engage your dog in scent work activities, such as hiding treats around the house for them to find.

Rest:

- Nap Time: Allow your dog time to rest and nap during the midday. Australian Shepherds, like all dogs, need downtime to recharge.

Afternoon Routine

Exercise:

- Afternoon Walk: Take your dog for another walk in the afternoon. This helps maintain their energy levels and provides additional mental stimulation.

- Off-Leash Play: If possible, visit a dog park or a secure area where your dog can run off-leash and socialize with other dogs.

Feeding:

- Lunch (Optional): Depending on your dog's dietary needs and feeding schedule, you may need to provide a small lunch or snack. Consult your veterinarian for personalized feeding recommendations.

Training:

- Training Session: Conduct another short training session to reinforce obedience commands and work on any behavioral issues. Consistent training helps maintain good behavior and mental sharpness.

Evening Routine

Potty Break:

- Evening Potty Break: Take your dog outside for an evening potty break before dinner. This helps prevent accidents and ensures they're comfortable.

Feeding:

- Dinner: Provide a balanced dinner that meets your dog's nutritional needs. Maintain consistency in meal times to create a predictable routine.

Exercise:

- Evening Walk: An evening walk helps your dog expend any remaining energy and promotes relaxation before bedtime. Keep the walk moderate in intensity.

Calm Activities:

- Relaxation: Engage in calm activities such as gentle play, cuddling, or brushing. This helps your dog wind down and prepares them for sleep.
- Potty Break: Take your dog out for a final potty break before bed.

Bedtime:

- Consistent Bedtime: Establish a regular bedtime to ensure your dog gets enough rest. Create a comfortable sleeping area that is quiet and free from disturbances.

Importance of Consistency

Consistency is crucial in building a routine for your Australian Shepherd. A predictable schedule provides several benefits:

1. **Security and Comfort:**
   - Predictable Environment: Dogs thrive in predictable environments. Knowing what to expect reduces

anxiety and helps your dog feel secure and comfortable.

- Trust and Bonding: Consistent routines foster trust and strengthen the bond between you and your dog.

2. Behavior Management:

- Good Behavior: Consistent schedules help reinforce good behavior by setting clear expectations and boundaries.
- Reducing Unwanted Behavior: Regular exercise and mental stimulation reduce the likelihood of destructive behaviors, such as chewing, digging, or excessive barking.

3. Health and Well-Being:

- Regular Exercise: Consistent exercise routines promote physical health, prevent obesity, and support overall well-being.

- Dietary Health: Regular feeding times help maintain a healthy metabolism and prevent digestive issues.

Adjusting to Changes

Life changes, such as moving to a new home or experiencing significant transitions, can disrupt your dog's routine. Here's how to help your Australian Shepherd adjust to changes smoothly:

Handling Moves and New Environments

Preparation:

- Familiarization: Before the move, familiarize your dog with packing materials and boxes. Allow them to explore these items to reduce anxiety.
- Gradual Introduction: If possible, gradually introduce your dog to the new

home or environment. Bring them for short visits before the actual move.

Consistency:

- Maintain Routine: Try to maintain as much of their existing routine as possible during the move. Stick to regular feeding, exercise, and bedtime schedules.
- Comfort Items: Bring along familiar items such as their bed, toys, and blankets to provide comfort in the new environment.

Exploration:

- New Environment: Allow your dog to explore their new home gradually. Start with one room and slowly expand their access to other areas.
- Supervision: Supervise your dog closely during the initial days in the new environment to ensure they feel safe and secure.

Coping with Life Changes

Significant Life Changes:
- Routine Disruptions: Life events such as the arrival of a new family member, changes in work schedules, or illness can disrupt your dog's routine.
- Adaptation Period: Allow your dog time to adapt to these changes. Maintain as much consistency as possible and gradually introduce new elements to their routine.

Managing Stress:
- Calming Techniques: Use calming techniques, such as providing a quiet space, using calming sprays, or offering comfort items, to help your dog manage stress.
- Extra Attention: Spend extra time with your dog, providing reassurance and comfort during times of change.

Professional Support:

- Training Assistance: If your dog struggles to adapt to changes, consider seeking help from a professional dog trainer or behaviorist.
- Veterinary Advice: Consult your veterinarian if your dog exhibits signs of severe anxiety or stress. They can provide guidance and recommend appropriate interventions.

Building a consistent and balanced routine is essential for the well-being of your Australian Shepherd. By establishing a structured daily schedule that includes feeding, exercise, training, play, grooming, and rest, you provide your dog with the stability and security they need to thrive. Consistency in routines helps manage behavior, promotes health, and strengthens the bond between you and your dog. When life changes occur, careful planning and gradual adjustments can help your dog adapt smoothly, ensuring they remain happy and well-adjusted throughout their life.

Chapter 12

Training for Specific Activities

Service and Therapy Training

Training your Australian Shepherd for specific activities such as service and therapy work can be an incredibly rewarding endeavor. These roles require specialized training to ensure the dog can perform necessary tasks reliably and behave appropriately in various environments. This chapter provides an in-depth guide on the basics of training a service dog, the process for therapy dog certification, and an introduction to canine sports and competition preparation.

Basics of Training a Service Dog

Service dogs are trained to perform specific tasks to assist individuals with disabilities. These tasks can range from physical support to alerting for medical conditions. Here's a detailed guide on the basics of training a service dog:

1. Understanding Legal Requirements:
- ADA Compliance: Service dogs must meet the standards set by the Americans with Disabilities Act (ADA). They are trained to perform specific tasks directly related to the handler's disability.
- Public Access Rights: Service dogs have legal access to public places where pets are generally not allowed, including restaurants, stores, and public transportation.

2. Selection of the Right Dog:
- Temperament Assessment: Not all dogs are suitable for service work. Ideal candidates are calm, confident, and highly trainable. Australian Shepherds can be excellent service dogs due to their intelligence and eagerness to please.

- Health Screening: Ensure the dog is in good health, with no genetic conditions that could impede their ability to perform tasks or live a long working life.

3. **Basic Obedience Training:**
   - Foundation Skills: Begin with basic obedience commands such as "sit," "stay," "come," "heel," and "down." These are the foundation for more advanced training.
   - Socialization: Expose the dog to a variety of environments, people, and other animals to ensure they remain calm and focused in different settings.

4. **Task-Specific Training:**
   - Task Identification: Identify the specific tasks the dog needs to perform based on the handler's disability. Examples include retrieving items, opening doors, alerting to sounds, or providing mobility support.
   - Step-by-Step Training: Break down each task into smaller steps and train them

incrementally. Use positive reinforcement techniques to encourage correct behaviors.

- Consistency: Ensure the dog can perform tasks reliably in various environments and under different conditions.

5. Public Access Training:

- Manners in Public: Train the dog to behave appropriately in public settings, including walking calmly on a leash, ignoring distractions, and remaining focused on the handler.
- Advanced Commands: Teach advanced commands such as "leave it," "watch me," and "under" (to tuck under tables or chairs).

6. Certification and Testing:

- Evaluation: While the ADA does not require certification, many handlers choose to have their service dogs evaluated by professional trainers or organizations to ensure they meet the necessary standards.

- Continued Training: Service dogs require ongoing training and reinforcement to maintain their skills and reliability.

Therapy Dog Certification

Therapy dogs provide comfort and support to people in hospitals, nursing homes, schools, and other facilities. Unlike service dogs, therapy dogs do not have public access rights but can visit specific places by invitation. Here's how to train and certify a therapy dog:

1. **Assessing Suitability:**
   - Temperament: Therapy dogs must be friendly, patient, and gentle. They should enjoy human interaction and be comfortable in various settings.
   - Behavior: The dog should have a calm demeanor, not easily startled or aggressive, and be well-behaved around people and other animals.

2. Basic Training and Socialization:

- Obedience Training: Start with basic commands such as "sit," "stay," "down," "come," and "leave it." The dog should respond reliably to commands.
- Socialization: Expose the dog to different environments, sounds, and people to ensure they are comfortable in various situations.

3. Advanced Training:

- Desensitization: Train the dog to be desensitized to medical equipment, loud noises, and sudden movements. They should remain calm in these environments.
- Interaction Skills: Teach the dog to interact gently with people, including those who may be frail or use medical equipment.

4. Therapy Dog Certification Process:

- Join a Therapy Dog Organization: Organizations such as the Alliance of

Therapy Dogs (ATD) and Therapy Dogs International (TDI) offer certification programs.

- Health and Temperament Test: The dog must pass a health examination and a temperament test to ensure they are suitable for therapy work.
- Training Evaluation: The organization will evaluate the dog's obedience and interaction skills. They may require the dog to perform specific tasks or demonstrate good behavior in simulated therapy settings.
- Supervised Visits: Some organizations require supervised visits to ensure the dog can perform well in real-life therapy situations.

5. Ongoing Training and Evaluation:

- Regular Training Sessions: Continue training sessions to reinforce good behavior and address any issues that may arise.

- Re-evaluation: Some organizations require periodic re-evaluations to ensure the dog maintains the necessary skills and temperament for therapy work.

Sports and Competitions

Engaging in canine sports and competitions can be a fantastic way to channel your Australian Shepherd's energy and intelligence. These activities provide physical exercise, mental stimulation, and strengthen the bond between you and your dog.

Introduction to Canine Sports

1. Types of Canine Sports:

- **Agility:** A fast-paced sport where dogs navigate through obstacle courses, including jumps, tunnels, weave poles, and more. It tests speed, coordination, and teamwork.
- **Obedience:** Dogs perform a series of predefined tasks, such as heeling, retrieving, and sitting or lying down at a

distance. It focuses on precision and control.

- Rally Obedience: A variation of traditional obedience with a course of signs indicating different commands. It emphasizes teamwork and communication.
- Herding: For breeds like Australian Shepherds, herding trials test their natural herding instincts and ability to manage livestock.
- Flyball: A relay race where dogs jump hurdles, trigger a box to release a ball, and return over the hurdles. It's a high-energy, team-oriented sport.
- Disc Dog: Dogs catch flying discs thrown by their handlers. It showcases athleticism, precision, and teamwork.
- Tracking: Dogs use their sense of smell to follow a scent trail. It simulates search and rescue scenarios and requires keen sensory skills.

2. Benefits of Canine Sports:

- Physical Exercise: Sports provide excellent physical exercise, helping to keep your dog healthy and fit.
- Mental Stimulation: Learning new skills and navigating challenges keeps your dog mentally sharp.
- Bonding: Working together in sports strengthens the bond between you and your dog, enhancing trust and communication.
- Socialization: Participating in sports exposes your dog to new environments, people, and other dogs, improving their social skills.

Preparing for Competitions

1. Choosing the Right Sport:

- Assess Your Dog's Interests and Abilities: Consider your dog's natural inclinations and physical capabilities. Australian Shepherds often excel in agility, herding, and obedience due to their intelligence and agility.

- Your Interests: Choose a sport that you find enjoyable and can commit to. Your enthusiasm and dedication are crucial for success.

2. Training for Competitions:

- Foundation Skills: Ensure your dog has solid obedience skills before advancing to sport-specific training. Basic commands and good manners are essential.

- Sport-Specific Training: Enroll in classes or work with a trainer experienced in your chosen sport. They can provide structured training and valuable insights.

- Gradual Progression: Start with basic elements of the sport and gradually increase difficulty as your dog becomes more proficient.

- Positive Reinforcement: Use treats, praise, and play to reward your dog's efforts and successes. Positive reinforcement builds enthusiasm and confidence.

3. Conditioning and Health:

- Physical Conditioning: Regular exercise and conditioning are important to prepare your dog for the physical demands of competition. Include a mix of endurance, strength, and flexibility exercises.
- Diet and Nutrition: Ensure your dog has a balanced diet to support their energy levels and overall health. Consult your veterinarian for specific dietary recommendations.
- Regular Vet Check-ups: Maintain regular veterinary check-ups to monitor your dog's health and address any issues early.

4. Mental Preparation:

- Exposure to Competition Environments: Familiarize your dog with the competition setting. Attend events as spectators to acclimate your dog to the sights, sounds, and atmosphere.

- Practice Runs: Simulate competition conditions during training to build confidence and reduce anxiety. Practice with distractions and varying environments.

5. Entering Competitions:

- Registering for Events: Find competitions through local clubs, organizations, and online resources. Register in advance and understand the rules and requirements.
- Trial Runs: Participate in practice trials or fun matches to gain experience without the pressure of official competition.
- Stay Calm and Positive: Your dog can pick up on your emotions. Stay calm, positive, and supportive to help your dog perform their best.

6. Sportsmanship and Etiquette:

- Respect: Show respect for judges, fellow competitors, and their dogs. Good sportsmanship enhances the experience for everyone.
- Learning from Experience: Win or lose, each competition is a learning opportunity. Celebrate successes and identify areas for improvement.

Engaging in service and therapy training, as well as canine sports, not only utilizes the exceptional abilities of your Australian Shepherd but also strengthens your bond and provides fulfilling activities for both of you. Whether assisting in essential tasks, providing comfort to those in need, or excelling in sports competitions, your Australian Shepherd can thrive and find joy in these specialized roles.

Chapter 13

Community and Support

Finding Support Groups

Connecting with other dog owners and enthusiasts can provide valuable support, advice, and camaraderie. This chapter explores various avenues for finding community and support for Australian Shepherd owners, including local dog clubs, online communities, and professional assistance.

Joining Local Dog Clubs

Local dog clubs offer opportunities to meet fellow Australian Shepherd owners, participate in events and activities, and access resources and support. Here's how to find and join a local dog club:

1. Research: Use online resources, community bulletin boards, and social media to search for dog clubs in your area.

2. Visit Meetings and Events: Attend club meetings, events, and activities to meet members and learn more about the club's focus and offerings.

3. Participate: Get involved in club activities such as training classes, breed-specific events, and community service projects.

4. Build Relationships: Form friendships and connections with other members who share your passion for Australian Shepherds.

Online Communities and Resources

The internet provides a wealth of resources and communities for Australian Shepherd owners. Here are some ways to find support and information online:

1. Social Media: Join Australian Shepherd-specific groups on platforms like Facebook, Reddit, and Instagram. These groups

often provide a forum for sharing photos, stories, and advice.

2. Forums and Discussion Boards: Participate in online forums and discussion boards dedicated to Australian Shepherds. Websites like AussieInfoNet and AussieManiacs offer platforms for asking questions, sharing experiences, and connecting with other owners.

3. Breed Clubs and Associations: Explore websites and online resources provided by Australian Shepherd breed clubs and associations. These organizations often offer educational materials, breed-specific information, and networking opportunities.

4. Blogs and Websites: Follow blogs and websites dedicated to Australian Shepherds for tips, training advice, and breed-related content. Look for reputable sources with accurate information and experienced authors.

Professional Help

When faced with challenges or seeking guidance on training, behavior, or health issues, professional assistance can be invaluable. This section covers when to consult a trainer and the importance of working with a veterinarian.

When to Consult a Trainer

Professional dog trainers can provide guidance, support, and expertise to address a wide range of training and behavior issues. Here are some situations where consulting a trainer may be beneficial:

1. Basic Obedience Training: If you're struggling with basic obedience training or need help teaching your Australian Shepherd essential commands.

2. Behavior Problems: If your dog exhibits behavioral issues such as aggression, fearfulness, separation anxiety, or excessive barking.

3. Specific Training Needs: If you're training your Australian Shepherd for specialized activities such as service work, therapy work, or competitive sports.

4. Puppy Training: If you're a first-time puppy owner and need guidance on socialization, house training, and basic manners.

5. Group Classes vs. Private Sessions: Consider whether group classes or private training sessions would be more suitable for your needs and preferences.

Working with a Veterinarian

Regular veterinary care is essential for maintaining your Australian Shepherd's health and well-being. Here's how to establish a positive relationship with your veterinarian:

1. Wellness Exams: Schedule regular wellness exams to monitor your dog's overall health and detect any potential issues early.

2. Vaccinations and Preventative Care: Follow your veterinarian's recommendations for

vaccinations, parasite control, and preventative care.

3. Nutrition and Diet: Consult your veterinarian for guidance on selecting the right diet and nutrition plan for your Australian Shepherd's age, breed, and health needs.

4. Health Concerns: If you notice any changes in your dog's behavior, appetite, energy level, or physical condition, consult your veterinarian promptly.

5. Emergency Care: Be aware of emergency veterinary services in your area and know when to seek immediate medical attention for your dog.

By connecting with supportive communities, seeking professional assistance when needed, and prioritizing regular veterinary care, you can provide the best possible care and support for your Australian Shepherd.

Chapter 14

Addressing Myths and Misconceptions

Common Myths about Australian Shepherds

Australian Shepherds, like many popular dog breeds, are surrounded by myths and misconceptions. In this chapter, we'll explore some of the most prevalent myths about Australian Shepherds and debunk them with accurate information and insights.

Debunking Breed Stereotypes

Myth 1: Australian Shepherds Need Acres of Space to Run:

Reality: While Australian Shepherds are energetic and enjoy physical activity, they don't necessarily require acres of space to thrive. With regular exercise, mental stimulation, and interactive play, Australian Shepherds can adapt well to various living environments, including apartments, as long as their exercise needs are met.

Myth 2: Australian Shepherds are Only for Experienced Dog Owners:

Reality: While Australian Shepherds are intelligent and active dogs that require proper training and socialization, they are not inherently difficult to handle. With patience, consistency, and a commitment to meeting their needs, Australian Shepherds can make wonderful companions for owners of all experience levels.

Myth 3: Australian Shepherds are Naturally Aggressive:

Reality: Australian Shepherds are not inherently aggressive. Like any breed, individual temperament varies, but with proper socialization, training, and responsible ownership, Australian Shepherds are typically friendly, affectionate, and well-mannered dogs.

Understanding True Breed Characteristics

What to Expect from Your Dog

To understand Australian Shepherds fully, it's essential to recognize their true breed characteristics:

1. Intelligence:

    Reality: Australian Shepherds are incredibly intelligent and thrive on mental stimulation. They excel in obedience training, agility, and problem-solving tasks.

2. Energy and Activity Level:

    Reality: Australian Shepherds are high-energy dogs that require plenty of physical exercise and mental stimulation to prevent boredom and behavioral issues. Daily walks, play sessions, and interactive games are essential for keeping them happy and healthy.

3. Herding Instincts:

Reality: Australian Shepherds have strong herding instincts, which may manifest as nipping, circling, or herding behavior towards people or other animals. Channeling these instincts through appropriate training and activities is crucial.

4. Loyalty and Affection:

Reality: Australian Shepherds form deep bonds with their families and are known for their loyalty and affectionate nature. They thrive on companionship and enjoy being actively involved in family activities.

Setting Realistic Expectations

Balancing Expectations with Reality

Setting realistic expectations is key to a harmonious relationship with your Australian Shepherd. Here's how to balance expectations with reality:

1. **Exercise Needs:**
   - Expectation: Australian Shepherds have high exercise needs and require daily physical activity to thrive.
   - Reality: Be prepared to commit to regular exercise and mental stimulation to keep your Australian Shepherd happy and healthy.

2. **Training Requirements:**
   - Expectation: Australian Shepherds are intelligent and trainable dogs.

- Reality: While Australian Shepherds are quick learners, they can also be independent and strong-willed. Consistent training, positive reinforcement, and patience are necessary for success.

3. **Socialization**:
   - Expectation: Australian Shepherds are typically friendly and social dogs.
   - Reality: Early and ongoing socialization is crucial to ensure your Australian Shepherd is well-mannered and confident around people, animals, and different environments.

4. **Time and Commitment:**
   - Expectation: Australian Shepherds require time, attention, and commitment from their owners.
   - Reality: Be prepared to invest time and effort into meeting your Australian Shepherd's physical, mental, and emotional needs. They thrive on

companionship and involvement in family life.

By understanding the true breed characteristics of Australian Shepherds and setting realistic expectations, you can build a strong, fulfilling relationship with your dog based on mutual understanding, respect, and companionship. With patience, consistency, and love, you'll enjoy the rewards of sharing your life with this remarkable breed.

Chapter 15

Celebrating Life with Your Australian Shepherd

Creating Lasting Memories

Celebrating life with your Australian Shepherd is about cherishing every moment you share together. From the everyday adventures to the extraordinary milestones, creating lasting memories ensures that the bond you share with your furry companion grows stronger with each passing day.

Fun Activities to Do Together

Engaging in fun activities with your Australian Shepherd strengthens your bond and creates unforgettable experiences. Whether exploring the great outdoors, participating in canine sports, or simply enjoying quality time at home, these activities provide joy and fulfillment for both you and your dog.

Capturing Special Moments

Capturing special moments with your Australian Shepherd allows you to preserve precious memories that you can cherish for years to come. Through photographs, videos, and keepsakes, you can immortalize the unique bond you share and relive cherished moments whenever you desire.

Lifelong Learning and Growth

Continuing education and training are essential components of celebrating life with your Australian Shepherd. Lifelong learning fosters growth, strengthens your bond, and enriches your relationship with your dog, ensuring that you both continue to evolve and thrive together.

Continuing Education and Training

Investing in continuing education and training for your Australian Shepherd is an ongoing commitment to their well-being and development. Whether honing existing skills or exploring new activities, continued learning fosters mental stimulation, physical fitness, and behavioral enrichment for your dog.

Embracing the Journey with Your Dog

Embracing the journey with your Australian Shepherd is about embracing every moment, overcoming challenges, and celebrating achievements together. Through the ups and downs of life, your dog remains a constant source of love, companionship, and unwavering loyalty, making every step of the journey worthwhile.

In celebrating life with your Australian Shepherd, you embark on a journey filled with love, laughter, and unforgettable memories. Through fun activities, special moments, ongoing learning, and unconditional devotion, you and your furry companion create a bond that transcends time and enriches your lives in countless ways.

Conclusion

Your Journey Ahead

As you reflect on your training journey with your Australian Shepherd, it's essential to celebrate the progress you've made and look forward to the future with optimism and enthusiasm. Your dedication, patience, and love have laid the foundation for a strong, fulfilling bond with your furry companion, and the journey ahead is filled with endless possibilities for growth and adventure.

Reflecting on Your Training Journey

Take a moment to reflect on the milestones you've achieved and the challenges you've overcome during your training journey with your Australian Shepherd. From mastering basic commands to tackling advanced skills, each step of the way has been an opportunity for learning, growth, and bonding with your dog.

Celebrating Progress

Celebrate the progress you've made together with your Australian Shepherd. Whether it's conquering a difficult behavior, achieving a training goal, or simply enjoying moments of joy and companionship, every milestone is a testament to your commitment and dedication as a dog owner.

Looking Forward to the Future

As you look forward to the future with your Australian Shepherd, embrace the endless possibilities that lie ahead. Whether it's embarking on new training adventures, exploring different activities together, or simply enjoying the journey of life, the bond you share with your dog will continue to deepen and evolve over time.

Resources for Continued Learning

To support your ongoing growth and development as a dog owner, consider exploring additional resources for continued learning and enrichment.

From recommended reading materials to helpful tools and online resources, there are countless ways to stay informed, engaged, and inspired on your journey with your Australian Shepherd.

Recommended Reading and Tools

- Books: Explore a variety of books on dog training, behavior, and care to deepen your understanding of your Australian Shepherd and enhance your training techniques.
- Online Courses: Consider enrolling in online courses or workshops to expand your knowledge and skills in areas such as obedience training, agility, or canine sports.
- Training Tools: Invest in high-quality training tools and equipment, such as leashes, harnesses, and interactive toys, to support your training efforts and provide mental and physical stimulation for your dog.

<u>Staying Informed and Engaged</u>

Stay informed and engaged in the dog community by connecting with other owners, trainers, and enthusiasts. Join local dog clubs, attend training classes or workshops, and participate in online forums and social media groups to share experiences, ask questions, and stay up-to-date on the latest trends and developments in dog training and care.

As you continue your journey with your Australian Shepherd, remember to cherish every moment, embrace every challenge, and celebrate every achievement along the way. With love, patience, and dedication, you and your furry companion can look forward to a lifetime of happiness, adventure, and shared memories together.

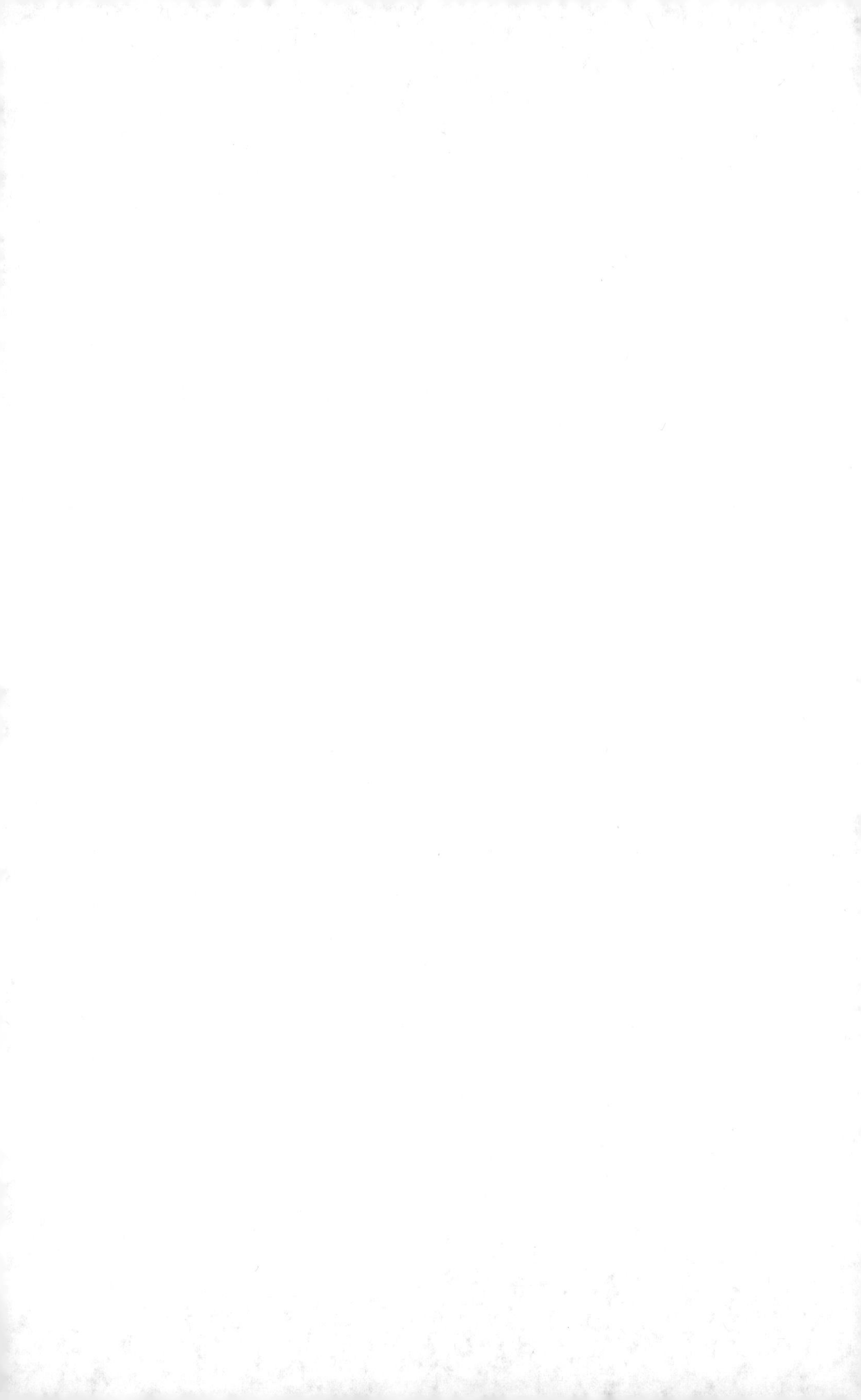

- Chew Toys: Chew toys or bones can help keep your dog occupied and reduce anxiety during the journey.

Calming Aids:

- Calming Sprays and Supplements: Use calming sprays, such as those containing pheromones, or natural supplements like CBD oil or chamomile to help reduce travel anxiety. Consult your veterinarian before using any calming aids.
- Anti-Anxiety Medications: In severe cases, your veterinarian may prescribe anti-anxiety medications to help your dog remain calm during travel. Use these medications as directed and test them before a long trip to ensure they are effective and well-tolerated.

Vacationing Together

Vacationing with your Australian Shepherd can be a wonderful adventure. Planning ahead and choosing dog-friendly destinations ensure a smooth and enjoyable trip for both of you.

Dog-Friendly Destinations

Researching Locations:
- Dog-Friendly Accommodations: Look for hotels, motels, vacation rentals, and campgrounds that welcome dogs. Many accommodations offer special amenities for pets, such as dog beds, treats, and designated play areas.
- Outdoor Activities: Choose destinations that offer plenty of outdoor activities suitable for dogs, such as hiking trails, dog parks, beaches, and lakes.

City Breaks:
- Urban Exploration: Many cities have dog-friendly parks, restaurants, and attractions. Research dog-friendly spots in the city you plan to visit and make a list of places where your dog will be welcome.

- Public Transport: Check the rules and regulations regarding dogs on public transport in the city. Some cities allow dogs on buses, trains, and trams, provided they are leashed or in a carrier.

Nature Getaways:
- National and State Parks: Many national and state parks have dog-friendly trails and campgrounds. Ensure you follow park regulations regarding leashing and waste disposal.
- Beaches and Lakes: Look for dog-friendly beaches and lakes where your Australian Shepherd can swim, run, and play. Always supervise your dog near water to ensure their safety.

Packing Essentials for Your Pet

Travel Gear:
- Leash and Harness: Bring a sturdy leash and a comfortable harness. A harness is

preferable for travel as it offers better control and is more secure.

- Crate or Carrier: If using a crate or carrier, ensure it is comfortable, well-ventilated, and appropriately sized for your dog.

Food and Water:

- Food Supply: Pack enough of your dog's regular food for the duration of the trip. Changing your dog's diet abruptly can cause digestive issues.
- Water: Bring plenty of fresh water and a portable water bowl. Hydration is crucial, especially during long trips and outdoor activities.

Health and Safety:

- Medical Records: Carry a copy of your dog's medical records, including vaccination history and any medications they are taking. This is important in case of emergencies.

- First Aid Kit: Pack a basic first aid kit for your dog, including bandages, antiseptic wipes, tweezers, and any necessary medications.
- Identification: Ensure your dog wears a collar with an ID tag that includes your contact information. Consider using a GPS tracker for added security.

Comfort Items:

- Bedding: Bring your dog's bed or a familiar blanket to provide comfort and a sense of home during the trip.
- Toys: Pack a selection of your dog's favorite toys to keep them entertained and comfortable.

Hygiene Supplies:

- Poop Bags: Bring an ample supply of poop bags to clean up after your dog during walks and outdoor activities.
- Grooming Supplies: Pack grooming essentials such as a brush, nail clippers,

and any necessary grooming products to keep your dog clean and well-groomed during the trip.